Strength Training
for Seniors Over 60

Most Effective exercises for elderly to
Improve Mobility and Balance

Dr. Bryant D Baldwin

Table Of Content

Strength exercises

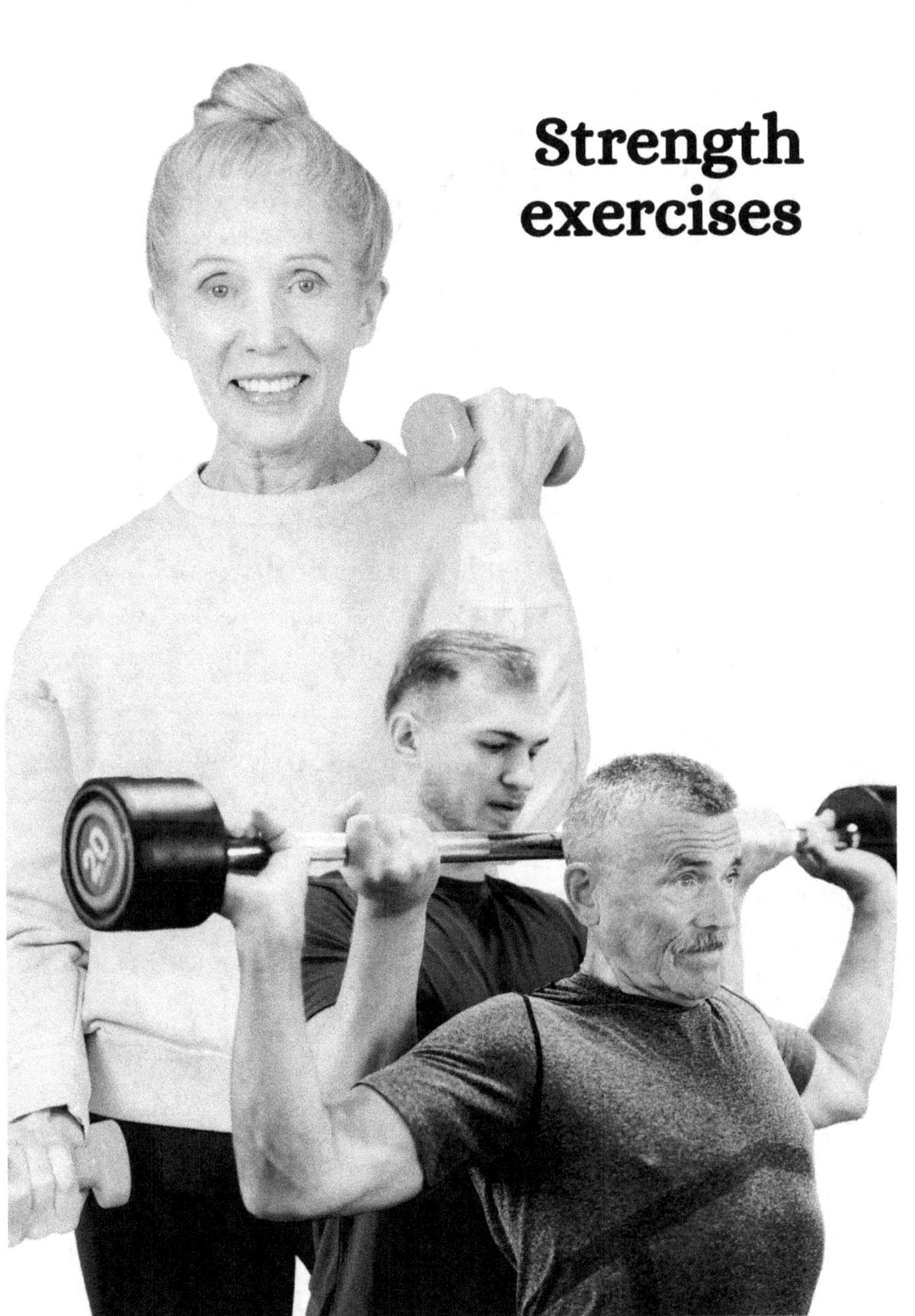

INTRODUCTION

As we age, preserving our physical health and well-being becomes increasingly crucial. One component that often goes forgotten, especially among seniors, is the need for strength training. While it's typical to identify strength training with younger persons or athletes, it is as vital for older adults to incorporate it into their workout regimens.

Strength training offers several benefits that can considerably improve the quality of life for seniors. It goes beyond just growing muscles; it helps raise bone density, improve balance and coordination, promote joint flexibility, and boost total functional fitness.

Engaging in regular strength-building exercises not only helps seniors execute daily activities with more ease and independence but also reduces the chance of falls and accidents, which can have major effects on this demographic.

Moreover, strength training has been found to have a good impact on numerous areas of seniors' health. It can assist control chronic illnesses such as arthritis, osteoporosis, and diabetes. It promotes cardiovascular health, boosts metabolism, and aids in weight management. Additionally, studies have revealed that strength training can have cognitive benefits, such as enhancing memory, concentration, and overall cognitive performance.

Despite the evident advantages, there are many misconceptions and concerns around strength training for seniors. One widespread fallacy is the worry of becoming harmed or overexerting oneself. However, with adequate coaching and a well-designed program, strength training may be both safe and effective for older persons. It's vital to recognize that strength training can be adapted to individual abilities, needs, and restrictions.

In this book, we will go into the area of strength training for seniors, exploring its benefits, addressing common misunderstandings and concerns, and providing practical help for getting started. We will emphasize the need for appropriate techniques, gradually increasing intensity, and the significance of working with healthcare specialists or fitness experts to guarantee a safe and tailored approach.

So, let's go on this journey of strength training for seniors and learn how it may improve your life, allowing you to age gracefully, keep independence, and live a bright and active existence for years to come.

The Benefits of Strength Training in Later Years

As we age, it becomes increasingly crucial to prioritize our physical well-being. One key part of keeping a healthy and active lifestyle in our later years is strength training. While many people connect strength training with younger folks or sports, it is equally (if not more) important for elders.

Strength training offers several benefits that can enhance the quality of life for older persons. By engaging in regular strength-building exercises, seniors can improve their muscle strength, increase bone density, and boost joint flexibility. These physical changes not only aid in doing daily duties more smoothly but also lower the chance of falls and injuries, which can be particularly problematic for seniors.

Furthermore, strength training has a significant impact on overall health and well-being. It helps to promote metabolism, regulate weight, and improve cardiovascular health. Additionally, studies have shown that strength exercise can boost cognitive function and mood, contributing to a sharper intellect and a more cheerful attitude toward life.

Overcoming Common Myths and Concerns

Despite the documented benefits of strength training for seniors, there are still frequent myths and worries that may dissuade persons from partaking in these activities. One popular myth is that strength training is only acceptable for younger, more physically fit persons. However, evidence indicates that seniors of varied fitness levels and abilities can safely and efficiently engage in strength training.

Another issue often voiced is the possibility of damage or strain. While it's vital to approach any new exercise plan with caution, when practiced correctly and under good instruction, strength training is generally safe for seniors. By learning the necessary techniques, using proper form, and gradually increasing intensity, the chance of damage can be minimized.

Importance of Consulting a Healthcare Professional

Before embarking on any new exercise regimen, elders need to check with a healthcare practitioner. They can provide tailored assistance, analyze any underlying health concerns or physical restrictions, and offer solutions appropriate to the individual's needs.

A healthcare practitioner may help build a strength training program that takes into account any pre-existing conditions or concerns, guaranteeing a safe and effective workout regimen.

How to Use This Book

This book strives to provide a thorough guide for seniors wishing to incorporate strength training into their lives. It will provide essential information, practical recommendations, and a selection of workouts ideal for varied fitness levels. Each chapter will focus on different areas of strength training, from knowing the principles to planning tailored exercises.

To get the most out of this book, it is recommended to read through each chapter consecutively. By following the progression, you will get a basic understanding of the principles and techniques involved in strength training for seniors. Additionally, the activities offered can be adjusted to your unique requirements and skills.

Remember, perseverance and patience are crucial when starting any new fitness adventure. With devotion and the knowledge presented in this book, you can experience the extraordinary benefits of strength training well into your elderly years.

Now, let's dig into the world of strength training for seniors and go on this revolutionary adventure together!

CHAPTER 1

Understanding Aging and exercise

In this chapter, we look into the interesting relationship between aging and exercise. As we journey through the natural process of aging, it becomes vital to comprehend the distinct changes our bodies undergo. By knowing how aging affects our physical capabilities and the role exercise plays in sustaining health, we may make informed choices for a meaningful and active existence. Get ready to examine the science behind aging and find the transforming impact of exercise in increasing vitality and well-being.

Age-Related Changes in Muscle Mass and Strength

With each passing year, our bodies undergo a loss in muscular mass, a condition known as sarcopenia. Starting as early as our 30s, this steady loss of muscle mass accelerates as we enter our senior years. Alongside lower muscle mass, there is also a decline in muscle strength and power, making it tougher to perform everyday activities and retain independence.

Multiple variables contribute to age-related changes in muscle mass and strength. Hormonal alterations, such as a drop in growth hormone and testosterone, have a role in muscle loss. Additionally, decreased physical activity, poor nutrition, and chronic health issues might further worsen these alterations. The combination of these causes creates a perfect storm, resulting in muscle degeneration and functional impairment.

Preserving Muscle Mass and Strength

While age-related changes in muscle mass and strength are unavoidable, there are proactive actions we can take to slow down the process and maintain optimal muscle health. The solution lies in adopting a holistic approach that involves exercise, good nutrition, and lifestyle improvements.

1. Resistance Training: Engaging in regular resistance training activities is vital for sustaining and increasing muscular mass. Strength training activities that entail lifting weights, utilizing resistance bands, or using body weight can stimulate muscular growth, improve strength, and boost general functional abilities.
2. Protein-Rich Diet: Adequate protein intake is needed for muscle maintenance and repair. Including lean meats, poultry, fish, dairy products, legumes, and plant-based protein sources in your diet can supply the required building blocks for muscle health.
3. Balanced Nutrition: A well-rounded diet, rich in fruits, vegetables, whole grains, and healthy fats, supplies the necessary nutrients, vitamins, and minerals to support general health and muscle performance. Additionally, being well-hydrated is crucial for good muscle performance.

4. Active Lifestyle: Leading an active lifestyle beyond structured exercise is vital. Incorporating activities such as walking, swimming, gardening, or dancing helps to retain mobility, improve circulation, and promote general well-being.

5. Adequate Rest and Recovery: Providing your muscles with enough rest and recovery time is vital for muscle growth and repair. Ensure you are receiving appropriate sleep and allowing for recovery intervals between workout sessions.

The Role of Exercise in Healthy Aging

Exercise is a magnificent weapon that can unleash the fountain of youth within us. Regular physical activity has been demonstrated to prevent the age-related reduction in muscle mass and strength, known as sarcopenia. By partaking in a well-designed exercise program, seniors can keep and even enhance their muscle mass, ultimately leading to greater mobility, balance, and independence.

Not only does exercise help in creating and maintaining muscle, but it also helps the general physiological functioning of the body. It contributes to enhancing bone density, joint flexibility, cardiovascular health, and metabolic function. Furthermore, exercise has been related to better cognitive capacities, emotional regulation, and a lower risk of chronic diseases such as diabetes, heart disease, and some malignancies.

Guidelines for Safe and Effective Exercise for Seniors

While exercise is a strong tool, it is vital to approach it with the correct understanding and supervision to guarantee safety and optimize its advantages. Here are some crucial suggestions for seniors wishing to embark on a safe and productive exercise routine:

1. Consult with a healthcare professional: Before starting any workout program, it is necessary to speak with a healthcare practitioner who can analyze your overall health, identify any

specific restrictions or considerations, and make individualized advice.

2. Focus on a well-rounded approach: Incorporate a variety of aerobic activities, strength training, balancing exercises, and flexibility routines to target different elements of fitness. This holistic strategy will assist maintain overall health, mobility, and functioning abilities.

3. Start gradually and progress slowly: Begin with easy workouts and progressively build intensity and length over time. This allows your body to adjust and decreases the danger of damage. Remember, calm and steady growth is crucial to long-term success.

4. Pay attention to good form and technique: It is vital to learn and practice good form and technique for each exercise to minimize strain or injury. Consider working with a certified fitness professional who can guide you in the correct execution of exercises.

5. Listen to your body: Tune in to your body's cues and alter your exercise plan accordingly. Rest when needed, and don't push past your boundaries. It's crucial to find the perfect balance between challenging yourself and respecting your body's capabilities.

Exercise is a valuable ally in the pursuit of good aging. By understanding the impact of age-related changes in muscle mass and strength, and executing a well-designed exercise program, seniors can effectively reverse the consequences of aging and enjoy a higher quality of life. The suggestions presented in this chapter serve as a path to safe and effective exercise for seniors, unlocking the potential for vitality, strength, and independence in the golden years. So lace up your sneakers, embrace the transformational power of exercise, and go on a journey towards a healthier, happier, and more fulfilled existence.

Essential Principles of Strength Training

Strength training is a dynamic and transforming discipline that goes beyond simply growing muscles. Whether you're a beginner or an experienced lifter, understanding the fundamental concepts of strength training is crucial for attaining optimal results and avoiding the risk of injury.

In this part, we look into the key ideas that constitute the core of good strength training programs. From progressive stress and good technique to individualization and recovery, we address the essential aspects that contribute to gaining strength, increasing muscle growth, and promoting overall fitness. Get ready to learn the secrets of successful strength training and go on a path toward a stronger, healthier you.

Importance of Proper Form and Technique

When it comes to strength training, proper form, and technique are not simply optional extras; they are crucial factors that can make or break your growth and entire training experience. Whether you are a beginner or an experienced lifter, recognizing the importance of perfect form and technique is crucial for maximizing results, reducing injuries, and ensuring long-term success. In this post, we will discuss the five essential reasons why excellent form and technique should be at the forefront of your strength training journey.

1. Maximizing Muscle Engagement and Targeting: One of the key reasons to stress appropriate form and technique is to ensure maximum muscle engagement and target the intended muscle groups effectively. By completing exercises with precise form, you work the targeted muscles to their utmost capacity, leading to optimal muscle development and strength improvements. Proper form also helps avoid the recruitment of compensatory muscles, ensuring that you're

predominantly engaging the intended muscle groups.

2. Preventing Injuries and Promoting Safety: Using good form and technique is vital for injury prevention and overall safety during strength training. When you execute exercises with improper form, you exert excessive stress on joints, tendons, and ligaments, increasing the risk of strains, sprains, and other injuries. Maintaining good alignment, managing the action, and avoiding unexpected jerks or excessive momentum lessen the likelihood of accidents and limit the wear and tear on your body.

3. Enhancing Performance and Efficiency: Proper form and technique go hand in hand with performance enhancement and efficiency in strength training. By completing exercises with precision, you increase movement efficiency and biomechanics, enabling you to lift bigger weights, complete more repetitions, and grow faster. When your body moves in a coordinated and efficient manner, you can generate more power and exertion, resulting in improved performance and better overall results.

Choosing the Right Equipment and Tools

Selecting the best equipment and tools for your strength training regimen is vital to fulfilling your unique goals and preferences. Consider the following variables while buying equipment:

1. Accessibility: Ensure that the equipment you chose is easily accessible and available for your workouts.
2. Versatility: Opt for equipment that allows you to execute a wide range of workouts and target numerous muscle groups.
3. Progression: Look for equipment that allows for progressive overload, enabling you to increase resistance over time as you get stronger.
4. Personal Preference: Consider your comfort level and satisfaction when utilizing different types of equipment, since it will help you stay motivated.

Planning Your Strength Training Program

Creating a well-structured and tailored strength training program is crucial to achieving continuous progress and optimal results. Consider the following tips when planning your program:

1. Goal Setting: Clearly define your goals, whether it's gaining muscle, increasing strength, improving sports performance, or enhancing general fitness.
2. Exercise Selection: Choose exercises that target all main muscle groups and employ a mix of complex (multi-joint) and isolation (single-joint) activities.
3. Training Frequency: Determine how many days per week you can spend on strength training, balancing it with other forms of exercise and recovery.
4. Progressive Overload: Gradually raise the resistance or intensity of your exercises to test your muscles and promote continual improvement.

Understanding Sets, Reps, and Intensity

Sets, repetitions, and intensity are important components that influence the volume and intensity of your strength training sessions. Consider the following aspects:

- Sets

A set is a series of consecutive repetitions of an exercise. Beginners may start with 1-3 sets for each exercise, while more proficient folks can perform 3-5 sets.

- Reps

Reps refer to the number of times you do a given exercise within a set. Higher reps (8-12) are commonly employed for muscular hypertrophy, while lower reps (1-6) are typically utilized for strength increases.

- Intensity

Intensity refers to the level of effort or resistance applied during a workout. It can be adjusted through elements like weight, resistance, or speed of movement. Choose an intensity that challenges you without losing perfect form.

CHAPTER 2

Warm-up and Cool-down Routines for Seniors

Keeping strength and mobility becomes increasingly crucial for overall health and well-being. For seniors, including warm-up and cool-down routines in their strength training regimen can be a game-changer. These vital preparatory and recovery phases not only optimize performance but also assist prevent injuries and promote longevity in physical exercise.

In this chapter, we will delve into the relevance of warm-up and cool-down routines specifically geared toward seniors looking to gain strength. We will investigate the benefits of these routines, discuss the specific exercises and techniques involved, and provide suggestions on how to combine them into a comprehensive training program. By learning and applying proper warm-up and cool-down procedures, seniors can unlock their full potential, boost their strength-building initiatives, and sustain an active lifestyle for years to come.

The Benefits of Warm-up Exercises

Warm-up exercises give a range of advantages that boost performance and prepare the body for physical activity. Here are five significant benefits:

1. Increased Blood Flow and Oxygen Delivery: Warm-up exercises enhance the body's core temperature, increasing blood flow and oxygen supply to the muscles. This primes the muscles for enhanced performance and minimizes the risk of damage.
2. Enhanced Joint Lubrication and Flexibility: Warm-up activities encourage the formation of synovial fluid, which lubricates the joints, reducing friction and stiffness. This, in turn, promotes joint flexibility and range of motion, allowing for safer and more effective movements during strength training.

3. Activation of Muscles: Warm-up activities engage and activate the muscles, preparing them for the approaching burden. This activation enhances muscle recruitment and coordination, resulting in enhanced muscular performance and total strength development.

4. Improved Neuromuscular Connection: Warm-up exercises facilitate the communication between the nerve system and muscles. This increased neuromuscular connection promotes muscle control, reaction time, and general coordination, minimizing the likelihood of falls or accidents while training.

5. Mental Preparation and Focus: Warm-up exercises also serve as a mental shift, letting seniors focus their attention on the impending workout. This mental readiness promotes concentration, motivation, and overall enjoyment of the strength training session.

Dynamic Warm-up Routine for Seniors

A dynamic warm-up program for seniors mixes gentle, yet effective, motions to prepare the body for strength training. Here are four exercises to include:

1. **Joint Rotations**

Begin with gentle joint rotations for the neck, shoulders, wrists, hips, knees, and ankles. This helps promote joint mobility and lubrication.

2. **Marching in position**

Lift your knees high while marching in position. This heats the lower body, boosts heart rate, and stimulates blood circulation.

3. **Arm Circles**

Stand tall and spread your arms out to the sides. Perform controlled circles with your arms, progressively increasing the range of motion. This workout warms up the shoulders and upper body.

4. **Leg Swings**

Stand near a wall or support and swing one leg forward and backward in a controlled manner.

This dynamic workout warms up the hips, hamstrings, and quads.

Cooling Down and Stretching Exercises

After completing the strength training program, cooling down and stretching activities are crucial for increasing recovery and flexibility. Here are some exercises to incorporate:

1. Standing Quad Stretch

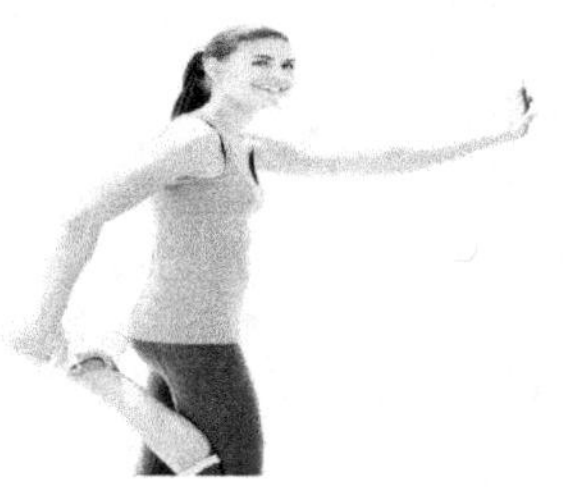

Stand tall and grasp onto a firm surface for balance. Bend one leg at the knee and grab your foot or ankle, moving your heel towards your glutes. Hold for 20-30 seconds on each leg to stretch the quadriceps.

2. Chest Stretch

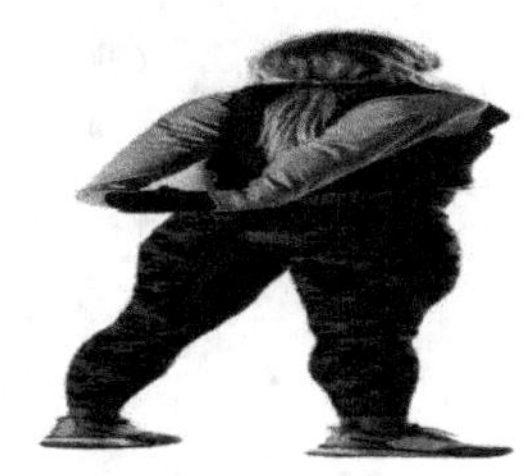

Interlace your fingers behind your back and gently straighten your arms while elevating your chest. This stretch targets the chest muscles and promotes improved posture.

3. Standing Calf Stretch

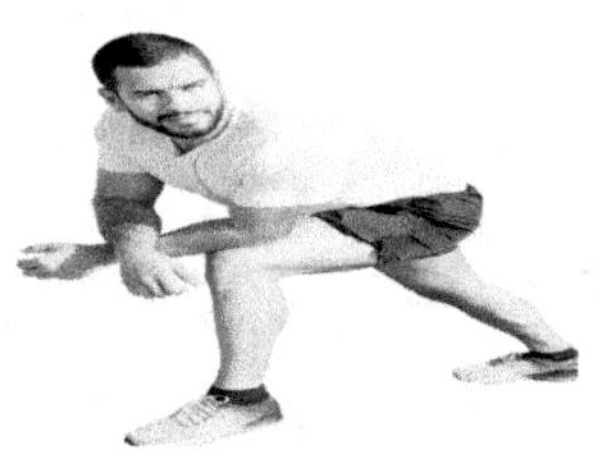

Stand facing a wall and place one foot a few feet behind the other. Lean forward, keeping your rear leg straight and heel on the ground, until you feel a stretch in your calf muscles. Hold for 20-30 seconds on each leg.

Integrating warm-up activities to prepare the body and mind for strength training and combining cooling down and stretching exercises for optimum recovery are vital components of a senior's strength-building journey.

By knowing and practicing these exercises, seniors can reap the benefits of greater performance, reduced chance of accidents, enhanced flexibility, and general well-being. Let us embrace the power of warm-up and cool-down routines, ensuring that every step towards gaining strength is conducted with safety, intention, and longevity in mind.

Upper Body Strength Exercises

Maintaining upper body strength becomes vital for keeping independence, improving posture, and enhancing the general quality of life. Seniors over 60 can harness the potential of specific workouts designed to strengthen their upper body muscles, increase mobility, and boost functionality.

In this part, we look into several efficient and safe upper-body strength exercises created exclusively for seniors. From workouts targeting the shoulders, arms, chest, and back, to movements that increase grip strength and posture, we will examine a broad repertory of exercises that enable seniors to build upper body strength and enjoy the benefits of an active, independent lifestyle.

1. Sitting Dumbbell Press

The seated dumbbell press is an effective workout for developing the shoulders, arms, and upper back muscles. Sitting on a firm chair or bench, hold a dumbbell in each hand at shoulder

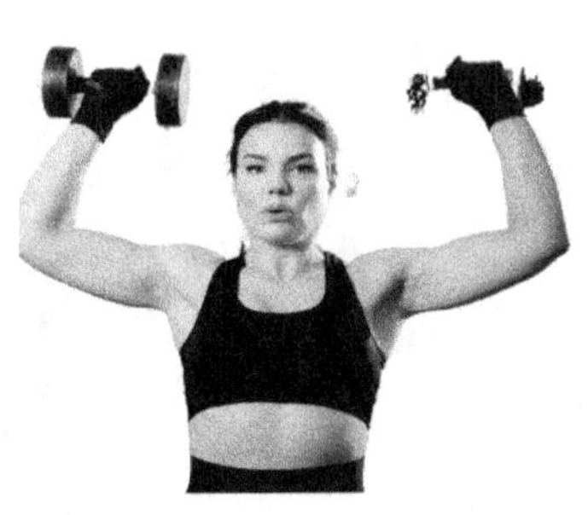

height. Press the weights overhead, completely extending your arms without locking the elbows. Lower the weights back down with control, keeping perfect form throughout the exercise. This exercise improves shoulder stability, promotes posture, and builds upper body strength.

2. Chest Press Machine

The chest press machine is an effective exercise for targeting the chest, shoulders, and triceps. Sit on the machine with your back on the padded backrest and grab the handles at chest level. Push the handles forward until your arms are

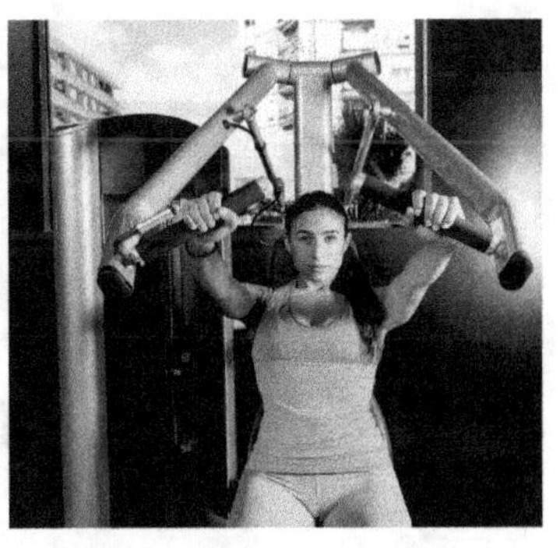

completely extended, then slowly return to the starting position. Focus on keeping appropriate form and controlled movement. The chest press machine strengthens the chest muscles, improves upper body pushing strength, and enhances total functional ability.

3. Seated Rows

Seated rows primarily target the muscles in the 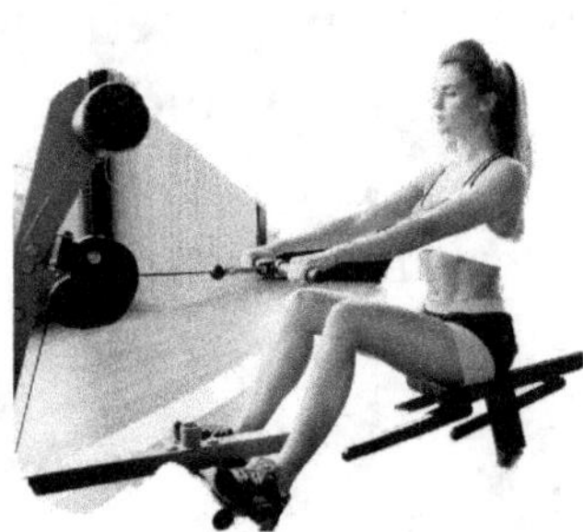 upper back, including the rhomboids, latissimus dorsi, and rear deltoids. Sit on a rowing machine with your feet firmly positioned on the footrests and your back straight. Grasp the handles with an overhand grip and draw them towards your body, pushing your shoulder blades together. Slowly remove the strain and extend your arms. Seated rows improve posture, strengthen the upper back muscles, and boost general back stability.

4. Bicep Curls with Resistance Bands

Bicep curls with resistance bands are a versatile and convenient workout for targeting the muscles in the front of the upper arms. Sit on a chair or bench with your feet firmly planted and

loop the resistance band under your feet. Hold
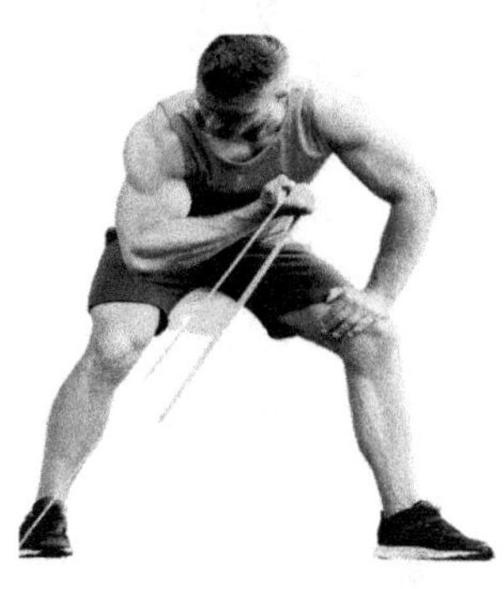
the ends of the band with an underhand grip, keeping your elbows close to your sides. Slowly curl your hands toward your shoulders, squeezing your biceps, and then lower the bands back down with control. This exercise builds arm strength, boosts grip, and supports activities that involve lifting and carrying.

5. Tricep Extensions

Tricep extensions effectively target the muscles at the rear of the upper arms. Sit on a chair or bench with your back straight and grip a dumbbell with both hands overhead. Slowly lower the weight behind your head by bending your elbows, then extend your
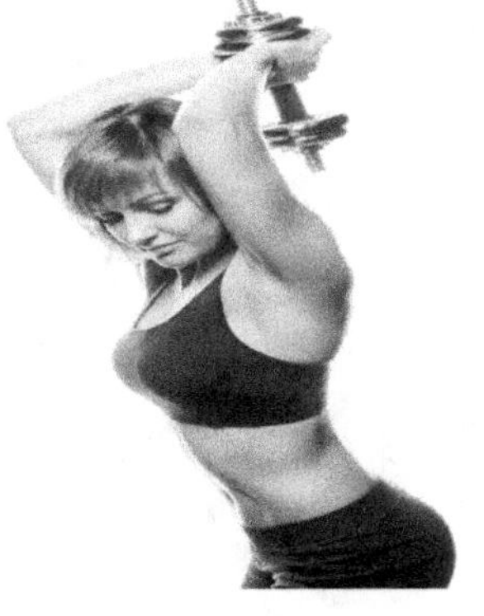
arms to raise the weight back up. Maintain

control during the action and avoid locking your elbows. Tricep extensions develop and tone the triceps, which assists in actions such as pushing, pulling, and reaching overhead.

Lower Body Strength Exercises

Maintaining lower body strength is critical for balance, stability, and independence. Engaging in specific workouts that focus on the lower body muscles can help seniors over 60 improve their mobility, prevent falls, and enhance overall functional capacity.

In this part, we explore a collection of effective and safe lower-body strength exercises designed exclusively for seniors. From squats and lunges to leg lifts and calf raises, we present a thorough guide to enable seniors to strengthen their lower body and enjoy the benefits of an active and confident lifestyle.

1. Leg Press

The leg press is a highly effective exercise for developing the quadriceps, hamstrings, and glutes. Sit on the leg press machine with your back on the backrest and your feet put on the footplate. Push against the footplate to stretch your legs, then progressively lower the weight

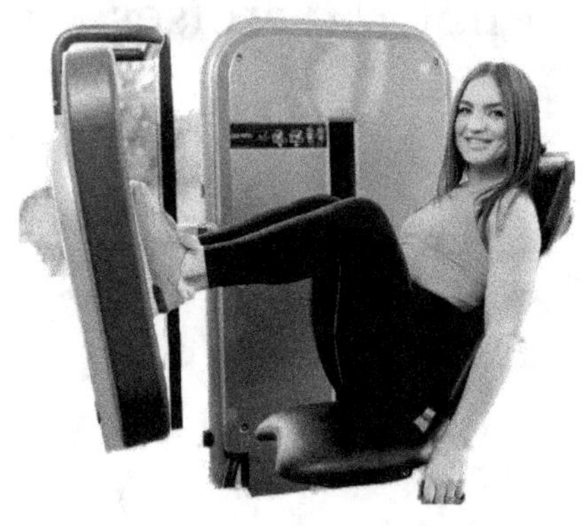

by bending your knees until they reach a 90-degree angle. Push the weight back up, completely extending your legs. The leg press builds lower body strength, enhances stability, and supports movements like walking, climbing stairs, and getting up from a chair.

2. Squats with Stability Ball

Squats with a stability ball are a safe and effective workout for developing the lower body, particularly the quadriceps, hamstrings, and glutes. Stand with your feet shoulder-width apart, placing a stability ball between your lower back and a wall. Keeping your back straight,

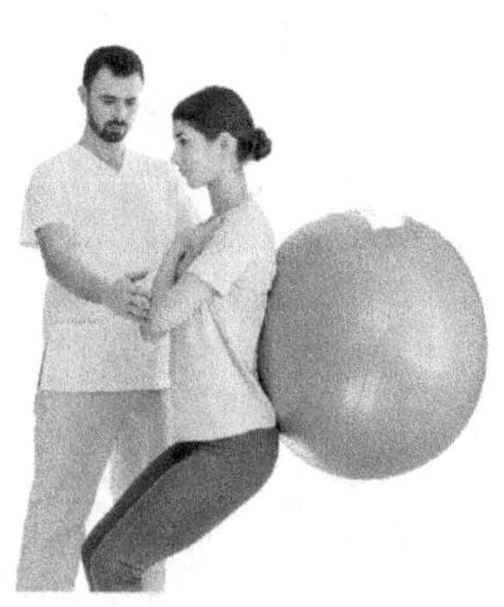

lower your body by bending your knees and hips as if sitting back in a chair. Ensure your knees stay aligned with your toes. Push through your heels to return to the starting position. Squats using a stability ball increase lower body strength, balance, and functional mobility.

3. Lunges with Dumbbells

Lunges with dumbbells target the quadriceps, hamstrings, glutes, and hip muscles. Stand tall with a dumbbell in each hand, step forward with

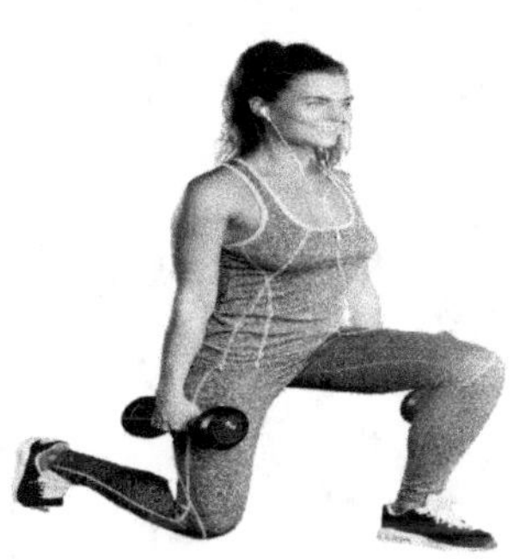

one leg, and lower your torso until both knees are at a 90-degree angle. Push back up to the starting position and repeat on the opposite leg. Lunges enhance leg strength, balance, and coordination, supporting actions like walking, climbing stairs, and maintaining equilibrium during daily motions.

4. Calf raises

Calf raises develop the calf muscles, which are vital for walking, balance, and stability. Stand with your feet hip-width apart, lift onto your toes, and hold for a moment before dropping your heels back down. For an added challenge, hold dumbbells in each hand. Calf raises can be performed on the floor or a raised platform like 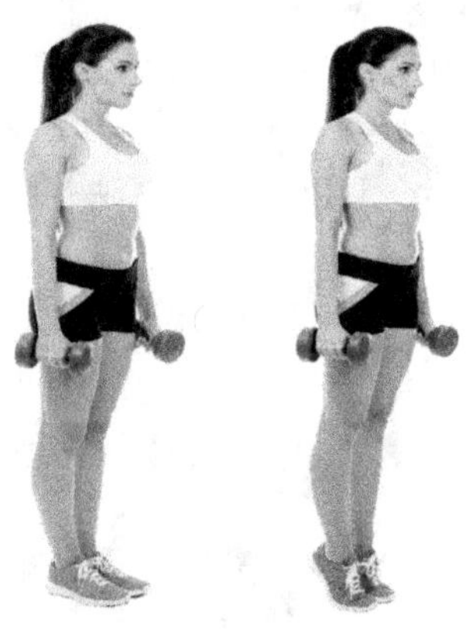 a step. This exercise builds calf strength, and ankle stability, and improves balance.

CHAPTER 3

Core and Balance Exercises

Core strength and balance maintenance becomes increasingly vital for overall stability, mobility, and confidence. Engaging in specific exercises that focus on the core muscles and improve balance can assist seniors over 60 strengthen their posture, reduce falls, and enjoy an active lifestyle with independence.

In this chapter, we delve into a selection of effective and safe core and balance exercises specifically created for seniors. From planks and seated twists to standing balance exercises and leg lifts, we will guide you through a thorough repertory of exercises that allow seniors to cultivate their core stability, enhance balance, and appreciate the benefits of a firm foundation.

Plank Variations

Planks are particularly effective workouts for developing the entire core, including the abdominal muscles, back muscles, and stabilizing muscles of the pelvis and hips. They also involve the upper body and lower body for increased stability.

Start by taking a push-up stance with your forearms resting on the ground, and elbows aligned beneath your shoulders. Keep your body in a straight line from head to toe, engage your core, and hold the position for a certain length. Plank variations might include side planks, forearm planks, and planks with leg lifts. These exercises strengthen core strength, improve stability, and support appropriate posture.

Seated Russian Twists: Seated Russian twists target the oblique muscles, which are necessary for rotational stability and total core strength. Sit on the floor with your knees bent, feet flat on the ground, and lean back gently while keeping proper posture. Hold a weight or medicine ball with both hands, stretch your arms in front of you, and spin your torso from side to side, touching the weight or ball to the ground on each side. Seated Russian twists strengthen core strength, enhance spinal mobility, and assist rotational movements.

Stability Ball Exercises for Core Strength

Stability balls are a diverse and efficient tool for increasing core strength and stability. Three key exercises include:

1. Stability Ball Crunches

Sit on the stability ball and walk your feet forward until your lower back is supported on 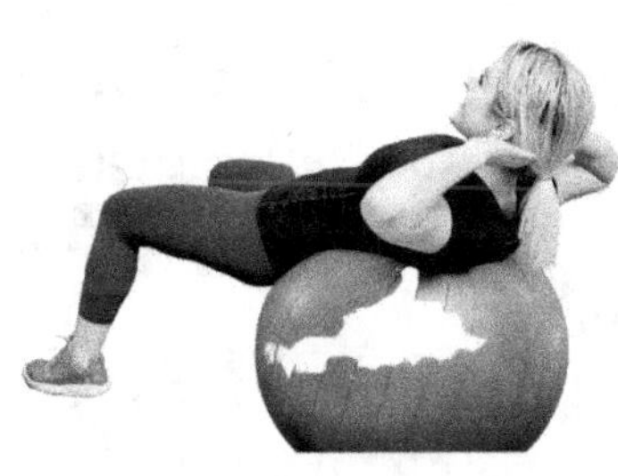 the ball. Cross your arms across your chest or place them behind your head. Engage your core and practice crunches by elevating your upper body towards your knees, then slowly drop back down. This workout targets the abdominal muscles and promotes core strength.

2. Stability Ball Plank

Place your forearms on the stability ball, elbows
aligned beneath your
shoulders, and extend
your legs out behind
you. Keep your body
in a straight line from
head to toe, engage
your core, and hold
the plank posture. This 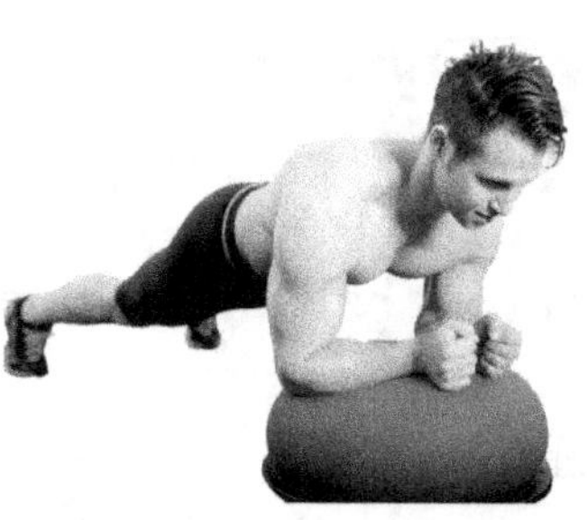
workout targets the core muscles and increases
stability.

3. Stability Ball Back Extensions

Lie face down on the stability ball with your
hips positioned at the center of the ball and your
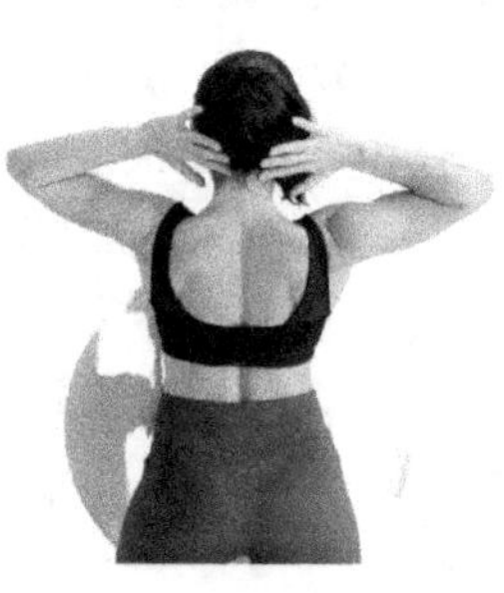 feet against a wall for
stability. Place your
hands behind your head
or cross them over your
chest. Engage your back
muscles and elevate your
upper body off the ball,
then slowly drop back
down. This exercise improves the back muscles
and encourages good posture.

Balance Exercises for Fall Prevention

Balance exercises are vital for seniors to increase stability, lower the risk of falls, and maintain independence. Three key exercises include:

1. Single Leg Stands

Stand near a sturdy surface and elevate one foot off the ground, balancing on the other leg. Hold the position for a set duration, then switch legs. This exercise improves balance and strengthens the leg muscles.

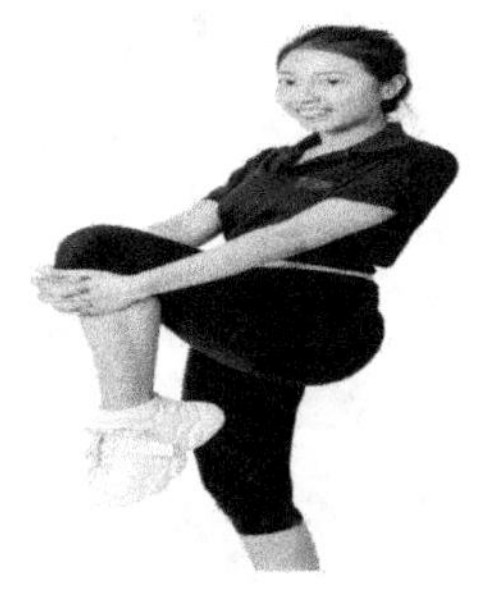

2. Heel-to-Toe Walk

Place one foot in front of the other, touching the heel of the forward foot to the toe of the back foot. Take modest steps in this heel-to-toe pattern, maintaining balance and coordination. This practice promotes proprioception and improves balance.

3. Standing Leg Lifts

Stand with feet hip-width apart and lift one leg
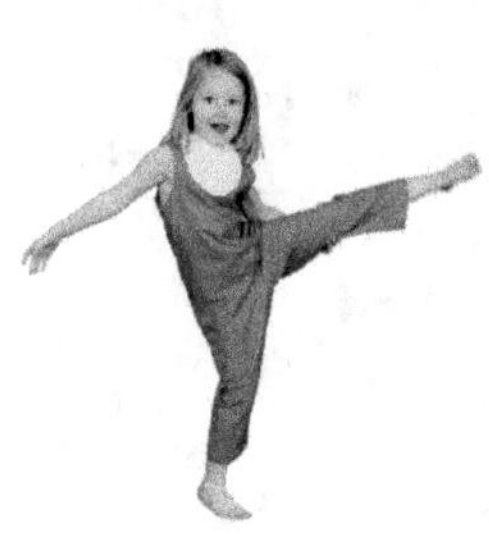
straight out in front of you
while keeping balance. Hold
the elevated leg for a moment,
then drop it back down.
Repeat on the opposing leg.
This exercise develops the leg
muscles and improves
stability.

Flexibility and Mobility Exercises

As we age, keeping flexibility and mobility becomes increasingly crucial for seniors over 60. Flexibility allows for a wide range of motion in joints, while mobility helps us to conduct daily activities with ease and elegance. Engaging in targeted exercises that focus on flexibility and mobility can help seniors better their general physical function, prevent injuries, and enjoy an active lifestyle with freedom and independence.

In this part, we delve into a range of efficient and safe flexibility and mobility exercises specifically created for seniors.

From mild stretches and range-of-motion exercises to dynamic motions and balance drills, we give a comprehensive guide to empower seniors to nurture flexibility, increase mobility, and appreciate the benefits of a flexible and nimble body.

Importance of Flexibility Training

Flexibility training offers a plethora of benefits for adults over 60. Here are four important reasons why including flexibility exercises in your workout program is crucial:

1. Improved Joint Range of Motion: Regular flexibility training helps preserve and even improve joint mobility, allowing seniors to use their limbs freely and comfortably. This boosts the ability to execute daily actions such as reaching, bending, and twisting with ease. Injury Prevention: Flexibility exercises assist improve muscular flexibility, minimizing the chance of strains, sprains, and muscle imbalances. By maintaining flexible muscles and tendons, seniors may navigate their daily lives with greater confidence and limit the chances of damage during physical activity.
2. Enhanced Posture and Alignment: Flexibility exercise promotes better posture and alignment by stretching tight muscles and releasing tension. Improved posture not only contributes to a more youthful appearance but also helps alleviate back discomfort and increases general body mechanics

3. Increased Functional Independence: Having adequate flexibility allows seniors to complete everyday chores independently, such as bending down to tie shoelaces, reaching for objects on high shelves, or getting in and out of chairs with ease. Flexibility training helps seniors to keep their functional independence and enjoy an active lifestyle.

Upper Body Stretches

Upper body stretches target the muscles in the arms, shoulders, chest, and back, encouraging flexibility and reducing stress. Some excellent upper body stretches for seniors include:

1. Overhead Triceps Stretch

Extend one arm overhead and bend it at the elbow, stretching your hand towards the opposite shoulder blade. Gently pull on the elbow with your other hand to deepen the stretch. This stretch targets the triceps muscle on the rear 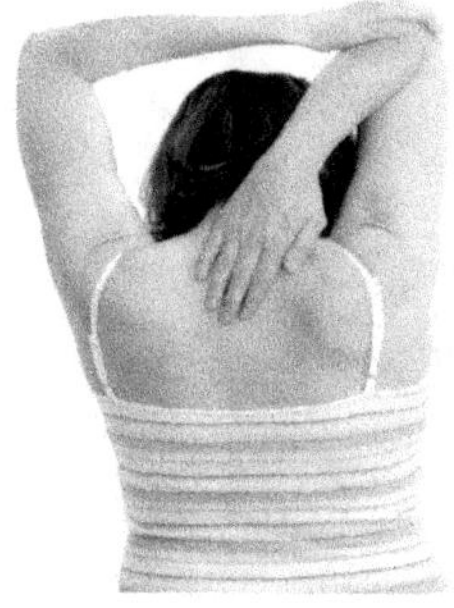 of the upper arm.

2. Shoulder Rolls

Stand tall with your arms relaxed by your sides. Slowly rotate your shoulders forward in a circular motion for numerous repetitions, then reverse the direction. This stretch helps reduce tension in the shoulders and promotes upper-body mobility.

3. Chest Stretch

Stand near a doorway and lay your forearm on the door frame with your elbow bent at a 90-degree angle. Gently lean forward until you feel a stretch in the chest muscles. Hold for a time, then switch arms. This stretch opens up the chest and counteracts the forward rounding of the shoulders.

Lower Body Stretches

Lower body stretches to focus on the muscles in the legs, hips, and lower back, encouraging flexibility and reducing tension. Some useful lower body stretches for seniors include:

1. Standing Quadriceps Stretch

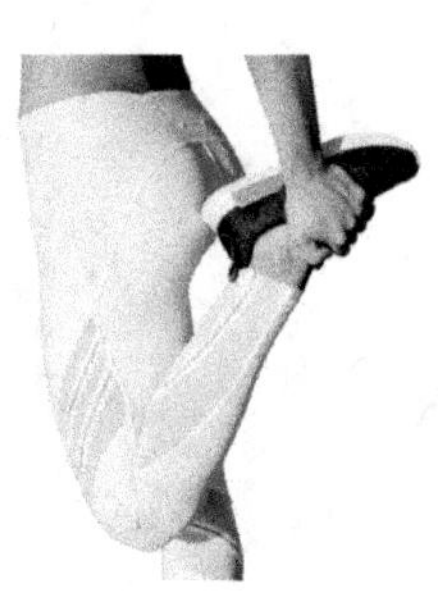

Stand tall, holding onto a sturdy surface if needed for balance. Bend one knee, bringing your foot towards your buttocks, and gently grip your ankle or use a strap or cloth to aid. Hold the stretch for a time, then repeat on the opposite leg. This stretch targets the quadriceps muscles at the front of the thigh.

2. Hamstring Stretch

Sit on the edge of a chair with one leg extended straight out in front of you. Keep your back straight and gradually extend towards your toes, feeling a stretch at the back of your thigh. Hold for a second, then swap legs. This stretch targets the hamstrings, which can get tight with age and inactivity.

3. Calf Stretch

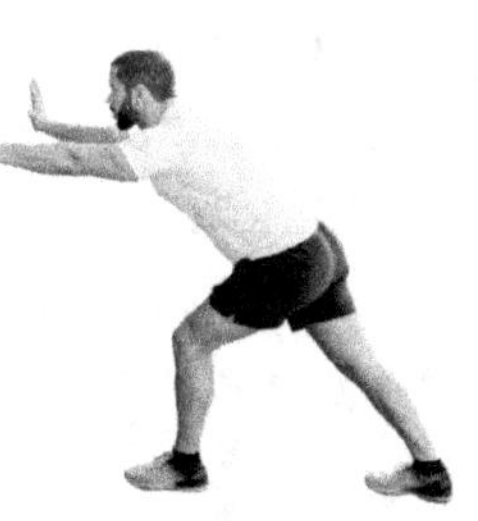

Stand near a wall or firm surface and place one foot forward, keeping the knee slightly bent. Lean forward, pressing your hands on the wall for support, and feel the stretch in your calf muscle. Hold for a second, then swap legs. This stretch focuses on the calf muscles, which play a critical role in balance and mobility.

Full-Body Mobility Exercises

Full-body mobility exercises focus on developing a general range of motion and joint mobility. These exercises frequently incorporate fluid motions and engage numerous muscle groups simultaneously. Some effective full-body mobility exercises for seniors include:

1. Standing March

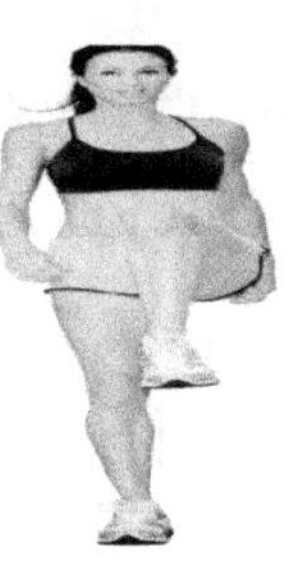

Stand tall with your feet hip-width apart and march in place, elevating your knees as high as comfortable. Swing your arms naturally to increase the flow of the movement. This exercise enhances flexibility in the hips and improves overall mobility.

2. Hip Circles

Stand with your feet hip-width apart and lay your hands on your

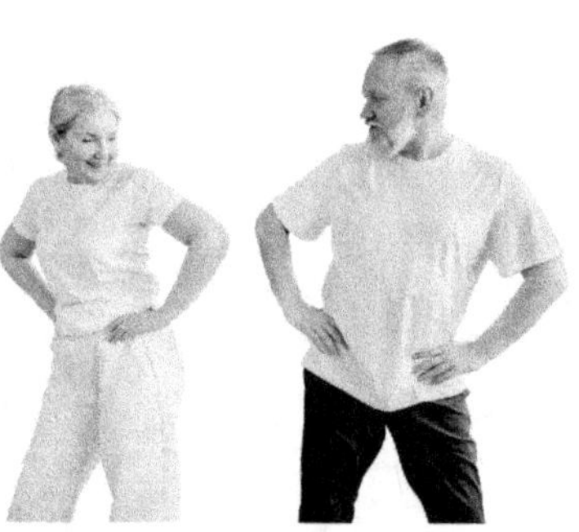

hips. Slowly rotate your hips in a circular motion, making smooth and controlled movements. This exercise helps enhance mobility in the hip joints and pelvic region.

3. Cat-Camel Stretch

Begin on all fours with your hands beneath your shoulders and knees beneath your hips. Arch your back upwards like a cat, tucking your chin 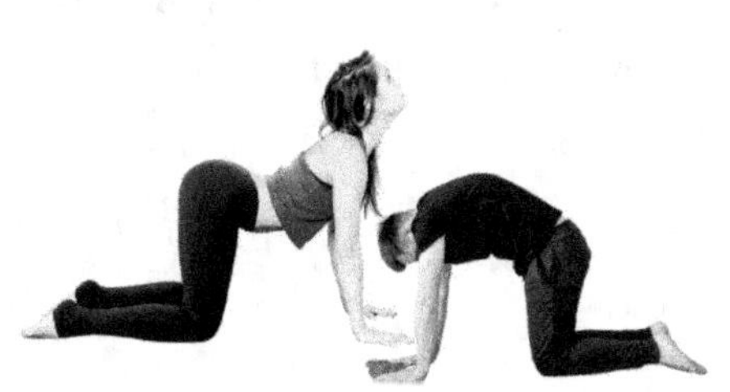 towards your chest, then slowly descend your belly towards the ground, raising your head and tailbone. Repeat this movement in a slow and controlled manner. The cat-camel stretch develops spinal flexibility and enhances movement throughout the entire spine.

CHAPTER 4

Designing Your Strength Training Program

Embarking on a strength training journey is a vital step towards developing your physical strength, enhancing your overall health, and enjoying a bright and active lifestyle. However, without a well-designed training program, your efforts may not deliver the expected results or, worse, lead to injuries or burnout.

In this chapter, we will cover the basic ideas and standards for developing a safe, effective, and tailored strength training program. Whether you are a beginner or have some expertise in strength training, understanding the fundamental components of program design can enable you to maximize your progress, optimize your performance, and unlock your maximum potential.

Designing a strength training program entails carefully selecting exercises, deciding proper sets and repetitions, modifying intensity levels, and considering issues like recovery and progression. It is a planned and strategic procedure that guarantees you reach your fitness goals while limiting the risk of injury and maintaining a balanced approach to training. By following the ideas mentioned in this chapter, you will be provided with the information and skills necessary to design a program that meets your needs, preferences, and talents.

Throughout this chapter, we will look into many components of designing your strength training program. We will study exercises that target different muscle groups, explain the notion of sets, repetitions, and intensity, and delve into topics such as equipment selection, scheduling, and measuring progress. Whether you aim to develop muscle, increase strength, improve overall fitness, or enhance sports performance, understanding the foundations of program planning is key to attaining success.

In addition to the technical aspects, we will also emphasize the significance of listening to your body, practicing appropriate form and technique, and incorporating flexibility and recovery into your training regimen. A well-rounded and sustainable approach to strength training involves not just testing your muscles but also nourishing them with care and allowing for proper rest and renewal.

As you continue on this chapter, remember that designing your strength training regimen is an ongoing process. It needs exploration, adaptability, and a willingness to learn from your body's response. With the information and assistance provided, you will be empowered to develop a program that coincides with your goals, talents, and lifestyle, unlocking your full potential and experiencing the transforming effects of strength training.

Setting Realistic Goals

Setting realistic goals is the core of every successful strength training program. Before going into your workouts, take the time to outline your objectives and determine what you aim to achieve. Whether your goals involve gaining muscle, boosting strength, strengthening endurance, or improving general fitness, it is vital to establish clear and attainable aims.

Realistic goals serve as a source of motivation, provide a sense of direction, and help you stay focused throughout your training journey.

Creating a Weekly Workout Schedule

A well-structured weekly workout schedule is a crucial component of a good strength training program. By selecting particular days and times for your workouts, you assure consistency and prioritize your training. Consider aspects such as your availability, energy levels, and other commitments while organizing your calendar. Aim for a fair distribution of workouts targeting different muscle groups, allowing for enough rest and recuperation between sessions.

Progression and Periodization Techniques

Progression and periodization are key techniques for continual growth and progress in strength training. Gradually increasing the demands placed on your muscles and challenging your body's limits is crucial to making growth. Incorporate progressive overload principles, such as increasing weights, repetitions, or intensity, to increase muscle adaptation and prevent plateauing.

Additionally, consider employing periodization strategies, which include alternating between different stages of training (e.g., hypertrophy, strength, power) to enhance performance and limit the risk of overtraining.

Incorporating Cardiovascular Exercise

While strength training is necessary for increasing muscle and strength, incorporating cardiovascular exercise is equally important for overall fitness and cardiovascular health. Including exercises such as brisk walking, jogging, cycling, or swimming in your workout program helps develop cardiovascular endurance, burn calories, and maintain a healthy heart.

Find a balance between strength training and cardiovascular activity that meets your goals and preferences, ensuring a well-rounded and complete approach to your fitness program.

Designing a strength training program takes careful consideration of different elements, from defining realistic goals to creating a weekly workout schedule, employing progression and periodization tactics, and combining cardiovascular activity.

By taking a careful and disciplined approach to program design, you can maximize your training, challenge yourself successfully, and feel the transforming advantages of strength training. Remember that building your program is a dynamic process that demands flexibility, adaption, and listening to your body's response. With the knowledge and ideas provided in this chapter, you have the skills to unlock your maximum potential and embark on a satisfying strength training adventure.

Safety Considerations and Modifications

Ensuring safety while strength training is of crucial importance, especially for seniors over 60. This chapter digs into critical safety considerations and adaptations targeted specifically for older persons. By learning good form, using suitable equipment, and adopting required adaptations, elders can enjoy the advantages of strength training while limiting the risk of injury. Embracing a safe and successful method will encourage seniors to embark on their fitness path with confidence and peace of mind.

Safety Tips for Seniors Engaging in Strength Training

Seniors should prioritize safety during strength training. Here are six crucial ideas to bear in mind:

1. Seek medical clearance: Consult with a healthcare expert before starting any workout

regimen, especially if you have pre-existing medical ailments or concerns.

2. Warm-up and cool down: Begin each session with a good warm-up to prepare your muscles and joints for activity, and end with a cool-down to aid in recovery.

3. Use good form and technique: Focus on maintaining perfect posture and executing exercises with proper form to avoid strain and lessen the risk of injury.

4. Start with lighter weights: Begin with lesser weights and progressively graduate to more challenging loads to guarantee optimal adaptation and reduce the danger of muscular strain.

5. Listen to your body: Pay attention to your body's messages and respect its limits. If you encounter pain or discomfort, alter your training or seek help from a certified specialist.

6. Stay hydrated and take breaks: Drink plenty of water before, during, and after your workouts. Take regular breaks to rest and recover as needed.

Modifying Exercises for Individual Needs and Limitations

Every individual has unique demands and limits. It is necessary to alter exercises adequately to accommodate these factors. Modifying workouts can involve modifying the range of motion, employing assistive equipment, or choosing alternate exercises that target the same muscle areas. By making proper adaptations, seniors can engage in strength training safely and efficiently, customizing the program to their skills and boosting their overall fitness.

Here are some major considerations for customizing exercises for individual requirements and limitations:

1. Range of Motion: Adjusting the range of motion is a typical alteration that can be advantageous for elders. If you have limited mobility or joint concerns, you can alter workouts to work within a comfortable range. For example, if practicing squats, you can utilize a chair for support, progressively decreasing the depth of the squat until you reach a range that suits your skills. By focusing on the

appropriate form and a controlled movement, you can still engage the target muscles efficiently while limiting the chance of discomfort or strain.

2. Assistive Devices: Using assistive devices can provide additional support and stability during strength training workouts. For example, if you have difficulties balancing during lunges or single-leg exercises, you might utilize a sturdy chair or wall for support. Resistance bands or straps can also be utilized to aid in doing certain workouts, such as bicep curls or tricep extensions. These gadgets can help maintain normal form and reduce the danger of falls or injury.

3. Alternative Exercises: In circumstances where some exercises are not suitable or provide obstacles owing to unique constraints, alternative exercises might be incorporated. For example, if regular push-ups are tough, modified push-ups against a wall or on an inclined surface can be performed to target the same muscle groups. The idea is to identify alternative exercises that target the same

muscle groups while taking into account your specific talents and limitations.

4. Adjusting Intensity: Modifying the intensity of workouts is vital for seniors to prevent overexertion and limit the chance of damage. This can be performed by altering the weight, repetitions, or sets. Start with lesser weights and progressively raise as you get more comfortable and stronger. It's vital to listen to your body and avoid straining beyond your boundaries. Working within a safe and reasonable level guarantees that you receive the advantages of strength training while limiting the danger of strain or overuse issues.

5. Incorporating Rest and Recovery: Rest and recovery are vital for seniors engaging in strength training. It's crucial to provide your body ample time to recover between sessions. If you encounter any discomfort or extreme muscular soreness, it's a hint that you may need to change your training schedule or allow for additional rest days. Adequate rest and recuperation assist prevent injuries and allow your body to adapt and strengthen in response to the activities.

Remember, it is always advisable to talk with a trained fitness professional or healthcare practitioner before starting a new workout program or making alterations. They can assist with your individual needs and restrictions, ensuring that your strength training program is safe and successful.

Common Injuries and How to Prevent Them

While engaging in strength training, it is vital to be aware of common injuries that can occur and adopt preventive precautions.

- Strains and Sprains

Muscle strains and ligament sprains are typical ailments that can develop from overexertion or incorrect technique during strength training.

To prevent strains and sprains, it is necessary to:

1. Warm up thoroughly before each session to prepare the muscles and joints for exercise.
2. Use good form and technique when conducting exercises, focusing on steady

movements and avoiding sudden jerking or twisting motions.

3. Start with lesser weights and gradually proceed to larger loads to allow muscles and connective tissues to adapt and strengthen.

4. Listen to your body and avoid straining beyond your limits, as weariness can increase the chance of injury.

5. Incorporate stretching exercises and flexibility training to maintain joint mobility and enhance muscle suppleness.

- Joint Discomfort

Joint discomforts, such as in the knees, hips, or shoulders, can arise owing to excessive stress or poor alignment during strength training. To prevent joint soreness, consider the following:

1. Choose exercises that are joint-friendly and do not exert excessive strain on sensitive areas.

2. Use suitable equipment and change settings to guarantee optimal alignment and reduce joint stress.

3. Incorporate workouts that strengthen the muscles around the joints, providing improved support and stability.
4. Focus on maintaining a balanced strength training program that stimulates both agonist and antagonist muscle groups, supporting joint stability and reducing muscle imbalances.
5. Avoid overtraining and provide appropriate rest and recuperation time between sessions to prevent overuse problems.

- Back Pain

Back pain can be a typical complaint among persons involved in strength training. To prevent back pain:

1. Prioritize core strength and stability exercises that assist support the spine and promote appropriate posture.
2. Use proper lifting techniques when handling weights or conducting activities that entail bending or lifting.

3. Engage the abdominal muscles and maintain a neutral spine throughout activities to prevent stress on the back.
4. Gradually increase the intensity and weight of workouts, allowing the back muscles and supporting systems to adjust.
5. Consult with a fitness professional or physical therapist to ensure you are completing exercises correctly and to obtain advice on necessary changes if needed.

CHAPTER 5

Nutrition and Recovery for Strength Training

Proper diet and recuperation play a critical part in maximizing the effects of strength exercise. Seniors over 60 who engage in strength training can enhance their outcomes by fuelling their bodies with the correct nutrition and giving ample time for recovery.

In this chapter, we will discuss the relevance of diet and recuperation in supporting strength training efforts and fostering general well-being. By knowing how diet affects muscle growth and repair and applying efficient recovery procedures, seniors can boost their performance, prevent injuries, and reach their fitness goals.

Importance of Proper Nutrition for Seniors

A proper diet is vital for elders engaging in strength exercise. Here are five main reasons why nutrition plays a crucial role:

1. Muscle growth and repair: Adequate protein consumption helps muscle growth and repair. It delivers the essential amino acids necessary to restore muscle tissues following strength training sessions, boosting overall strength and functionality.
2. Bone health: Seniors require sufficient calcium and vitamin D to sustain bone health and prevent age-related diseases like osteoporosis. A well-balanced diet rich in dairy products, leafy greens, and fortified foods can contribute to keeping strong and healthy bones.
3. Energy and performance: Proper nutrition ensures seniors have the required energy to do their strength training activities efficiently. A diet that combines complex carbohydrates, healthy fats, and lean proteins offers the fuel needed for optimal performance and endurance during workouts.

4. Immune system support: Nutrition plays a vital role in sustaining a robust immune system. A well-nourished body can better resist illnesses and infections, allowing seniors to maintain constant training and prevent setbacks.
5. Overall health and well-being: Proper diet contributes to overall health and well-being. It supports good weight management, helps regulate blood sugar levels, and reduces the risk of chronic diseases such as heart disease, diabetes, and certain types of cancer.

Hydration and nutrition Timing

Hydration and nutrition timing are key elements to consider for elders engaging in strength training. Proper hydration helps maintain normal bodily processes and supports performance throughout workouts. Seniors should attempt to consume water regularly throughout the day and during their exercise sessions to prevent dehydration.

Nutrient timing includes ingesting the proper nutrients at specific times to maximize their advantages. Seniors should attempt to take a balanced breakfast or snack comprising carbohydrates and protein within 1-2 hours following their strength exercise session. This helps refill energy storage, improves muscle regeneration, and aids in recuperation.

Rest and Recovery Strategies

Rest and recovery are as vital as the training itself. Seniors need to prioritize rest and recovery to allow their bodies to adapt, mend, and grow stronger. Here are some helpful rest and recuperation measures for seniors:

1. Sufficient sleep: Getting enough sleep is critical for muscle regeneration, hormone balance, and overall recovery. Seniors should aim for 7-9 hours of quality sleep each night.
2. Active recovery: Engaging in modest physical exercises such as gentle stretching, walking, or low-intensity aerobics on rest days can stimulate blood flow, reduce muscle soreness, and enhance recovery.
3. Proper stress management: Chronic stress can impair recuperation and hinder progress. Seniors could employ stress management techniques such as meditation, deep breathing exercises, or engaging in enjoyable hobbies to promote relaxation and healing.

4. Listening to the body: Seniors should pay attention to their bodies and adapt their training intensity or volume as needed. Pushing through extreme exhaustion or pain can raise the risk of injury and hinder recovery.
5. Incorporating rest days: Seniors should include regular rest days within their training program to allow for full recuperation. These rest days offer the body time to repair and regenerate muscular tissues, lowering the danger of overtraining and tiredness.

Proper nutrition, hydration, nutrient timing, and efficient rest and recovery measures are critical for seniors participating in strength exercise. By targeting these characteristics, older persons can boost their performance, promote muscle growth and regeneration, prevent injuries, and support their general health and well-being. It is crucial to speak with a healthcare practitioner or a certified dietitian for tailored nutrition recommendations and to ensure that any special dietary needs or limits are considered. By using these tactics, seniors can optimize their strength training efforts and enjoy the myriad benefits that come with an active and healthy lifestyle.

CONCLUSION

Frequently Asked questions

- Can I Start Strength Training in My Later Years?

Absolutely! It is never too late to start strength training. In reality, strength exercises can be incredibly useful for older folks. It helps increase muscle strength, bone density, balance, and overall functional ability. However, it is crucial to start cautiously and contact a healthcare practitioner before commencing any fitness regimen. They can provide assistance suited to your unique needs and ensure that you engage in safe and suitable workouts.

- How Often Should I Work Out?

The frequency of strength training activities will depend on several aspects such as your fitness level, overall health, and personal goals. In general, it is advisable to engage in strength training exercises at least two to three times per week. This allows for sufficient recuperation and muscle growth. It is crucial to have rest days between workouts to give your muscles time to recover and rebuild. Additionally, integrating other forms of exercise, such as cardiovascular activities, on alternate days can give a well-rounded fitness plan.

- What if I Have Joint Pain or Chronic Conditions?

If you have joint pain or chronic diseases, it is vital to contact a healthcare practitioner before commencing a strength training program. They can assess your condition and provide recommendations on exercises that are safe and suitable for your scenario. In some circumstances, adaptations or alternate workouts may be prescribed to accommodate joint limitations or address specific health issues. Working with a certified fitness professional or physical therapist who specializes in senior fitness can also be advantageous in establishing an activity program that takes your condition into account.

- Can Strength Training Help with Osteoporosis?

Yes, strength exercise can be incredibly beneficial for those with osteoporosis. Weight-bearing activities and resistance training can help enhance bone density and lower the incidence of fractures. However, it is vital to speak with a healthcare professional or a competent exercise specialist who can provide direction on appropriate exercises and adaptations unique to your condition. They can assist create a program that targets areas at risk for osteoporotic fractures, guaranteeing safety and effectiveness.

- How Long Will It Take to See Results?

The time it takes to see results from strength training might vary depending on various factors, including your starting point, frequency of exercises, intensity, and consistency. Generally, you may start feeling improvements in strength, balance, and mobility within a few weeks of consistent strength training. However, major gains in muscle strength and changes in body composition may take several months of persistent training. It is crucial to approach strength training with patience and a long-term view, as progress may vary for each individual. Remember that persistence and dedication to appropriate form and technique are crucial to getting the desired results over time.

Sample Strength Training Workout: Full-Body Routine

Warm-up: 5-10 minutes of light cardio, such as brisk walking or cycling, to stimulate blood flow and warm up the muscles.

Exercises:

- Squats: 3 sets of 10-12 repetitions

Stand with feet shoulder-width apart, and lower your body by bending the knees and pressing the hips back, maintaining the chest high and core engaged. Return to the starting location and repeat.

- Push-ups (Modified or Full): 3 sets of 8-10 repetitions

Place your hands on the floor shoulder-width apart (or on an elevated surface for a modified version). Lower your body by bending the elbows until your chest is near the ground, then push back up to the starting position.

- Seated Rows: 3 sets of 10-12 repetitions

Sit on a rowing machine or use resistance bands. Hold the handles with arms extended, then draw the handles towards your chest while pulling your shoulder blades together. Return to the starting location and repeat.

- Dumbbell Shoulder Press: 3 sets of 8-10 reps

Hold dumbbells at shoulder level, palms facing forward. Press the dumbbells above until your arms are fully stretched. Lower them back to shoulder level and repeat.

- Step-ups: 3 sets of 10-12 reps per leg

Stand in front of a step or platform. Step one foot onto the step, pressing through the heel, and raise the opposing leg. Step back down and repeat on the other leg.

- Plank: Hold for 30-60 seconds

Start in a push-up position, then descend onto your forearms. Keep your body in a straight line from head to toe, activating your core muscles. Hold this position for the appropriate duration.

Cooldown: 5-10 minutes of easy cardio, such as walking or cycling, followed by stretching activities for main muscle groups.

Note: This is simply a sample workout and should be modified based on individual fitness levels and any special constraints or advice from a healthcare practitioner or fitness trainer. It is vital to start with lesser weights and progressively increase intensity as strength and technique improve.

<u>My exercise log</u>

Activities			Time	Sets	Reps.

Activities			Time	Sets	Reps

Activities			Time	Sets	Reps

Senior Strength Training Plan

Warm-Up (5 minutes):
1. Cardiovascular Warm-Up:
   - Begin with 5 minutes of light aerobic activity like walking in place or stationary cycling to increase heart rate and warm up muscles.

Strength Training Routine (25 minutes):

2. Bodyweight Squats:
   - Stand with feet shoulder-width apart. Sit back and down as if sitting into a chair, then stand back up. Perform 2 sets of 12 reps.

3. Wall Push-Ups:
   - Stand facing a wall, arms extended at chest height. Perform push-ups against the wall. Aim for 2 sets of 10 reps.

4. Chair Leg Raises:
   - Sit on a sturdy chair, lift one leg straight out, then lower it without touching the floor. Alternate legs. Do 2 sets of 12 reps on each leg.

5. Seated Row:

- Sit on the edge of a chair, hold a resistance band in front, and pull the band towards your chest. Perform 2 sets of 15 reps.

6. Dumbbell Bicep Curls:

- Hold a lightweight dumbbell in each hand, palms facing forward. Curl the weights toward your shoulders. Aim for 2 sets of 12 reps.

7. Leg Press on a Stability Ball:

- Lie on your back with feet on a stability ball. Lift hips, then lower them back down. Perform 2 sets of 10 reps.

8. Dumbbell Shoulder Press:

- Sit or stand with dumbbells at shoulder height, press weights overhead. Do 2 sets of 12 reps.

9. Side Leg Raises:

- Stand beside a sturdy surface for support. Lift one leg to the side, then lower. Alternate legs. Perform 2 sets of 12 reps on each leg.

Cool Down (5 minutes):

10. Seated Chest Opener:
   - Sit tall, clasp hands behind your back, and open your chest. Hold for 30 seconds.

11. Triceps Stretch:
   - Bring one arm overhead, bending your elbow, and gently reach down your back with your opposite hand. Hold for 30 seconds on each arm.

12. Quad Stretch:
   - Stand, bringing one foot toward your buttocks and holding the ankle. Hold for 30 seconds on each leg.

Tips:
- Start with lighter weights and gradually increase as your strength improves.
- Perform exercises in a controlled manner, focusing on proper form.
- Include strength training 2-3 times per week with at least one day of rest between sessions.
- Consult with a healthcare professional before starting any new exercise routine.

This strength training plan is designed to enhance muscle strength and overall functional fitness for seniors. Adjust intensity based on individual capabilities and always prioritize safety during workouts.

Scan Here to join our 28 Day workout challenge